Integrating a Palliative Approach:
ESSENTIALS FOR PERSONAL SUPPORT WORKERS

WORKBOOK

Katherine Murray
RN, BSN, MA, CHPCN(C)

Life and Death Matters
Victoria, BC

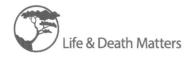
Life & Death Matters

www.lifeanddeathmatters.ca

Published by Life and Death Matters, Victoria, BC, Canada
www.lifeanddeathmatters.ca

Illustrations by Joanne Thomson
Editing by Sarah Weber
Design by Greg Glover

Library and Archives Canada Cataloguing in Publication

Murray, Katherine, 1957-, author
        Integrating a palliative approach. Workbook : essentials
for personal support workers / by Katherine Murray ; edited by
Sarah Weber ; illustrated by Joanne Thomson ; graphic design
by Greg Glover.

Supplement to: Integrating a palliative approach / Katherine
        Murray.
Includes bibliographical references and index.
Integrating a palliative approach.
ISBN 978-1-926923-05-5 (pbk.)

        1. Palliative treatment. 2. Terminal care. 3. Terminally ill--
Care. I. Title.

R726.8.M868 2014 Suppl.   616.02'9   C2014-906912-X

Disclaimer

This book is intended only as a resource of general education on the subject matter. Every effort has been made to en-
sure the accuracy of the information it contains; however, there is no guarantee that the information will remain current
beyond the date of publication. The information and techniques provided in this book should be used in consultation
with qualified medical health professionals and should not be considered a replacement, substitute, or alternative for
their guidance, assessment, or treatment. The author and publisher accept no responsibility or liability with respect to
any person or entity for loss or damage or any other problem caused or alleged to be caused directly or indirectly by
information contained in this book.

Contents

Reflective Writing: A Learning Practice

Our "baggage" is made up of the beliefs and values that each of us has learned and accumulated. Our baggage is reflected every day in our actions and words. In order to effectively meet the needs of dying people, you, as a personal support worker (PSW), must become aware of your own beliefs and values, and learn how to set them aside so they don't interfere with your ability to provide individualized care. When you become conscious of your beliefs and values, you can acknowledge them without imposing them on others.

Reflective writing is a way to identify and reflect on your own beliefs and values. This workbook will help you begin writing about them in a non-critical way. When you write, ignore spelling, grammar, and anything else that stops you. Avoid analyzing your writing. Your goal is to freely express yourself. Ignore the critic inside. Include drawings, write in point form or full sentences, and use coloured pens or pencils or anything else that helps you express yourself. You may need to reflect and write several times when thinking through an important topic. This is normal. The awareness that you gain from the writing is more important than what the writing looks like.

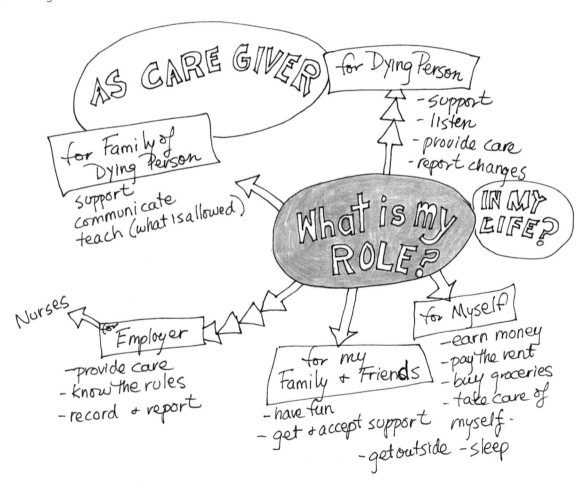

When you feel you have exhausted a topic, take a moment to read your response and reflect on it. It is okay to feel surprised, shocked, happy, sad, or any other emotion. These feelings are part of the reflective writing process. If your feelings are particularly strong, you may want to explore them further. This process of writing and reflecting will help you become aware of your own beliefs and values.

Later in the workbook, you are asked to write reflectively. You will be able to identify areas in which your current beliefs may get in the way of caregiving. Once you have identified them, you may want to spend time exploring where the beliefs came from and how they help or interfere with your ability to provide good care.

Choose a quiet and peaceful place for writing. Listen to your inner self, and enter into this practice with an open mind, prepared for self-discovery.

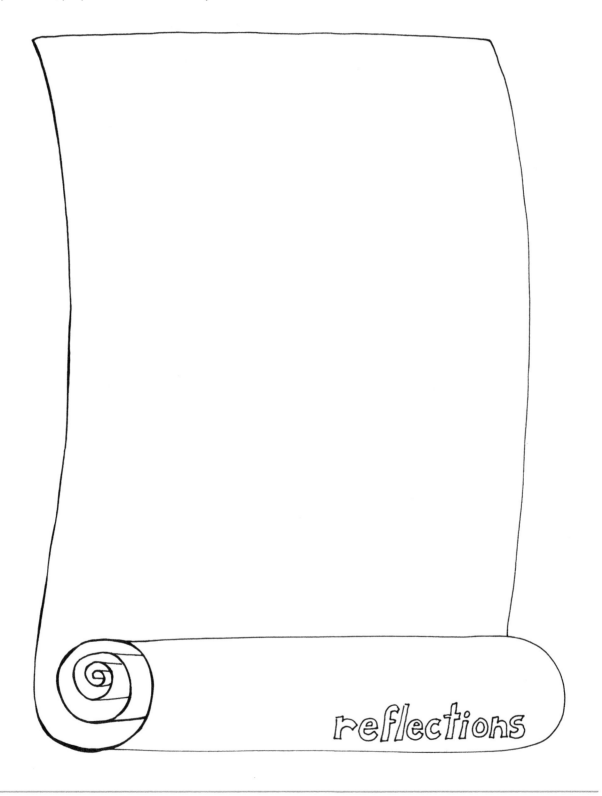

reflections

Preparing to Care

Understanding Your Beliefs and Baggage

1. What is self-awareness? How would you describe it, in your own words?

   _____

   _____

   _____

2. Identify an early experience you had related to death, dying, and/or grief.

   a. Describe the experience.

   _____

   _____

   _____

   b. What support did you receive?

   _____

   _____

   _____

   c. How did this experience affect you?

   _____

   _____

   _____

3. Circle the faces in the illustration below that reflect some of your feelings about working with people who are dying.

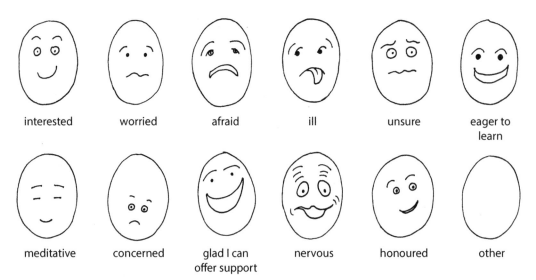

interested   worried   afraid   ill   unsure   eager to learn

meditative   concerned   glad I can offer support   nervous   honoured   other

4. Label the baggage in the illustration below with some of the beliefs and baggage related to death, dying, and/or grief that you carry with you to work. What beliefs and baggage will you need to put aside when caring for dying people?

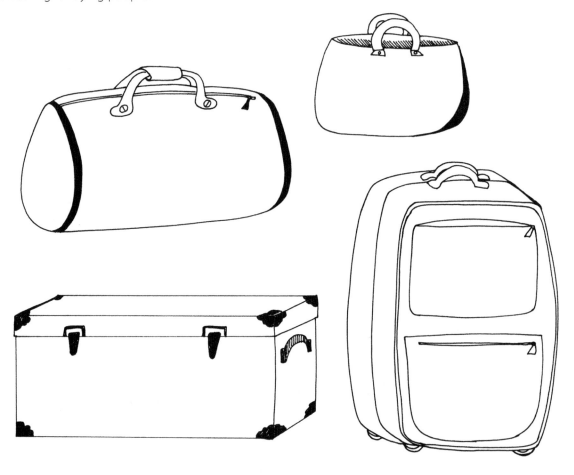

Solidifying Concepts

5. As discussed in the "Maintaining Therapeutic Boundaries" section on pages 6 to 10 in the text, therapeutic boundaries are necessary when providing care. Maintaining therapeutic boundaries is not always easy.

    a. How might you know if you are not maintaining boundaries?

        i. _____

        ii. _____

        iii. _____

    b. What steps can you take to establish therapeutic boundaries?

        i. _____

        ii. _____

        iii. _____

Integrating into Practice

6. In pairs or small groups, discuss the following:

    a. Similarities and differences between your definitions of self-awareness

    b. Experiences you have had related to death, dying, and/or grief

    c. Feelings you have about working with people who are dying

    d. The concept of baggage that you carry and the need to put baggage aside to care for others

7. In small groups, discuss the story about the homeless woman on page 5 in the text. Think about and share an experience you had when you judged someone. Describe the feeling you had about the person. Did your attitude toward them change when you learned more about them? If so, how did it change? What strategies can you use to help you learn not to judge or label people?

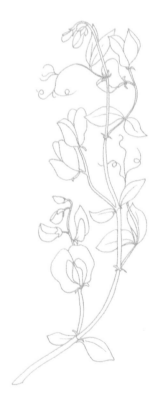

Understanding the Dying Process

2

Understanding Your Beliefs and Baggage

1. Think about the four different patterns of decline (trajectories) and place them in order of your most preferred ("good death") to least preferred ("bad death") way of dying. Draw and name each pattern on the "flip chart" provided. On the right-hand side of the chart, write two reasons why you placed them in the order you did.

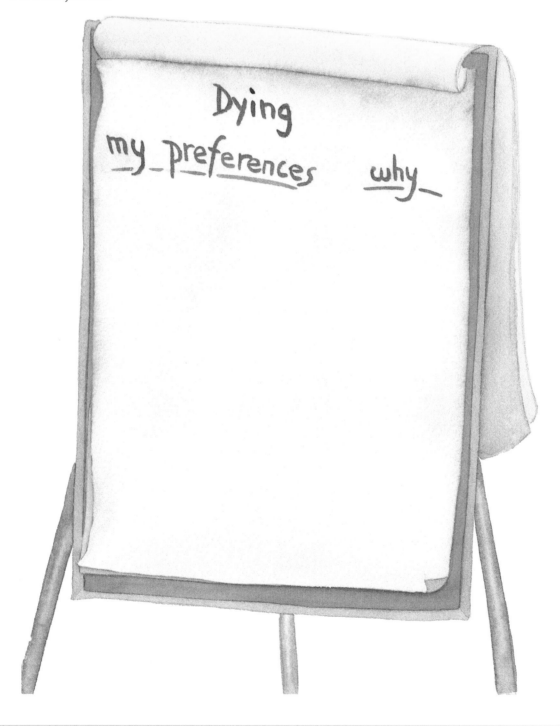

2. Reflect on the trajectory you would choose for a loved one.

    a. Which trajectory would you choose?

    _____

    _____

    _____

    b. Did you want something different for your loved one than you wanted for yourself?

    _____

    _____

    _____

    c. Is it harder or easier to imagine and choose a path for someone else? (Sometimes people find it more difficult to make decisions on behalf of another person. And people may choose more aggressive intervention for someone else than they would want for themselves.)

    _____

    _____

    _____

Solidifying Concepts

3. How is dying different today than it was in times gone by?

    a. _____

    b. _____

    c. _____

4. Review the stories of different patterns of decline in chapter 2 of the text. Complete the table below.

Pattern of decline	Impacts on the person	Impacts on the family	Ways that you as a PSW can support the person and the family
Steady decline	1. 2.	1. 2.	1. 2.
Stuttering decline	1. 2.	1. 2.	1. 2.
Slow decline	1. 2.	1. 2.	1. 2.

5. When they understand the unique challenges associated with each pattern or trajectory of dying , PSWs can best support the dying person and the family, and individualize care to meet the person's unique needs.

   a. Why do you think it is important to help a dying person maintain their ability to make choices as long as possible?

   _____

   _____

   b. List two strategies PSWs use to support a dying person to maintain choices.

   i. _____

   ii. _____

Integrating into Practice

6. It is important that you share information with the health care team about the dying person's preferences and goals of care. Reflect on what you would want your family and the health care team to know about you, if they needed to care for you when you were dying. For example, location, interventions, people present, level of medication and so on.

   _____

   _____

   _____

   _____

   _____

   _____

   _____

   _____

   _____

   _____

   _____

Integrating a Palliative Approach into Caregiving

3

Understanding Your Beliefs and Baggage

1. One key message of the text is that the principles of hospice palliative care can be integrated into care early in the dying process. Is this a new concept for you? Write about this idea. What are the benefits of the palliative approach? Do you already follow some of these principles?

_____

_____

_____

_____

_____

_____

2. Review pages 36 to 46 in chapter 3 of the text and identify good communication practices that you already use.

_____

_____

_____

_____

3. Recall a time when someone shared a painful experience with you and you wanted to help "fix" the problem. What part of your response suggests that you were in the Fix-It Trap?

_____

_____

_____

_____

_____

Solidifying Concepts

4. Complete the crossword puzzle on hospice palliative care below.

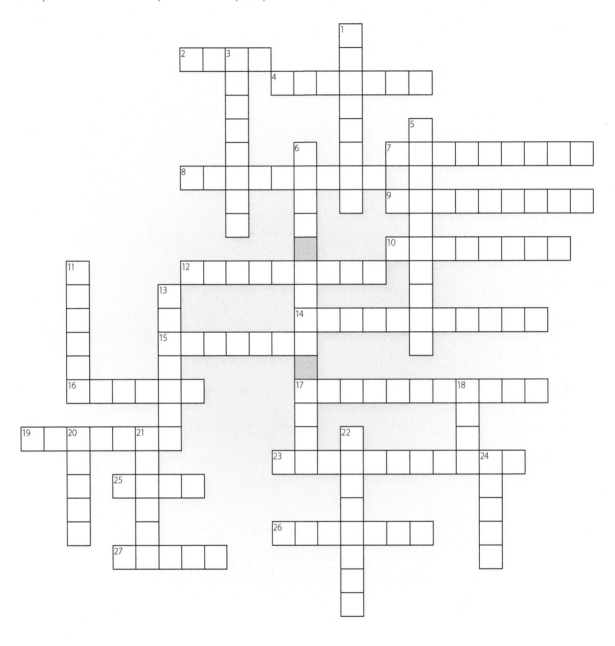

Across

2. HPC is best when provided by a _____.

4. HPC is known for improving a person's _____ of life.

7. A palliative approach is provided in many care settings, including home and _____ care.

8. A palliative approach can begin as early as _____.

9. _____ care, referring to the last weeks or months before death, lacks a standard definition. (3 words)

10. The founder of the first hospice in England was Dame _____.
12. A hospice society is an organization that offers services such as counselling and _____ support for the dying and bereaved.
14. An inpatient unit or home where a dying person can live their last weeks or months may be called a _____ hospice.
15. A primary goal of hospice care is _____ management.
16. HPC considers dying to be a _____ part of life.
17. When providing care for the dying person and the family, the PSW needs to _____ the person's needs to the care team.
19. _____ refers to a program of care provided for people whose prognosis (expected time of death) is less than six months and to the bereaved. It can also refer to the place providing care.
23. Care for the family continues through death and _____.
25. The patient and family are considered to be the _____ of care.
26. The practice of HPC _____ life.
27. People often need hospice support to deal with feelings of _____ and loss.

Down

1. Managing the needs of the entire person means looking at their _____ needs.
3. Applying the principles of HPC for any person with a life-threatening disease, early in the disease process, across all care settings, is referred to as "integrating a palliative _____."
5. At work, the PSW needs to maintain therapeutic _____.
6. The length of time people live in _____ is shorter now because people often arrive with multiple comorbidities. (3 words, with a space before and after the second word)
11. PSWs look and _____ to gather information on the needs of the dying person.
13. A palliative approach can be beneficial for symptom management for people in end-stage cardiac _____.
18. Individuals receiving hospice care often report better quality of life and greater satisfaction with _____.
20. The evolving _____ of practice of PSWs across Canada and the lack of consistency between facilities means that PSWs should review their roles and responsibilities with their employer.
21. The common belief that HPC is only for people with end-stage _____ and those in the last weeks or months of life is mistaken.
22. It is important to integrate a palliative approach across all care _____.
24. As a PSW, you will often report your findings to the _____.

(Answer key is on page 59.)

5. Using the text, define the following terms: hospice palliative care, end of life care. How are they the same? How are they different?

Hospice palliative care: _____

End of life care: _____

Differences: _____

Similarities: _____

6. List three principles of hospice palliative care.

_____

_____

_____

7. Circle the best definition of the palliative approach:

   a. The integration of hospice palliative care principles, practices, and philosophy into care for people with cancer, started in the last six months before death

   b. The integration of hospice palliative care principles, practices, and philosophy into care for people with all life-threatening illnesses, early in the disease process, across all care settings

   c. The integration of hospice palliative care principles, practices, and philosophy into care for people with all life-threatening illnesses, only in the last six months of life, in a hospice palliative care unit

8. Circle the best description of hospice palliative care:

   a. Regards dying as a normal process, considers the person and family as the unit of care, and continues through death and into bereavement

   b. Improves the quality of life, addresses holistic needs, and ends at time of death

9. Review pages 37 to 40 in the text and identify four common roadblocks to empathy and communication.

_____

_____

_____

_____

10. Identify whether the following statements express sympathy or empathy (circle your answer):

   a. I feel so sorry for you.   Sympathy   Empathy

   b. I hope you feel better soon.   Sympathy   Empathy

   c. I can hear the sadness in your voice even on the telephone. I am here for you if you want to talk about it.   Sympathy   Empathy

   d. I feel so badly that your mother died.   Sympathy   Empathy

   e. It sounds like you are overwhelmed with things to do. How can I help?   Sympathy   Empathy

Integrating into Practice

11. At work or during your practicum, talk with a member of the team and ask how hospice palliative care is provided to the people in their care.

12. Work in pairs. In the role-play described below, one participant will be Person A and the other will be Person B.

   a. Person A talks about a concern or a problem that they have. For example, "I am worried about the exam next week" or "My mom is sick and she may have cancer. My dad is also not well."

   b. Person B will respond with a roadblock to communication (see pages 37 to 40 in the text).

   c. Person A will consider their internal reaction to this type of response.

   d. Person B will consider how it felt to reply with a roadblock and observe the effect it had on Person A.

   e. Reverse your roles and observe your responses to roadblocks.

   f. Reverse the roles again, but this time ask open-ended questions. Consider how it felt to ask these questions, and how it felt to receive a question that helped to stimulate thinking, rather than a road-block.

   g. Discuss the exercise and identify ways to encourage communication.

13. Using the flip chart on page 17, brainstorm to create your own list of characteristics of what would be a good death and a bad death for you.

During class or with a partner, compare lists and answer these questions:

a. Did anyone's list surprise you?

_____

_____

b. How might you adapt care to help meet individual preferences?

_____

_____

_____

14. Refer to the "Dignity Question" on page 42 in the text. Then imagine that you are dying. What does the health care team need to know about you to give you the best care possible?

_____

_____

_____

_____

_____

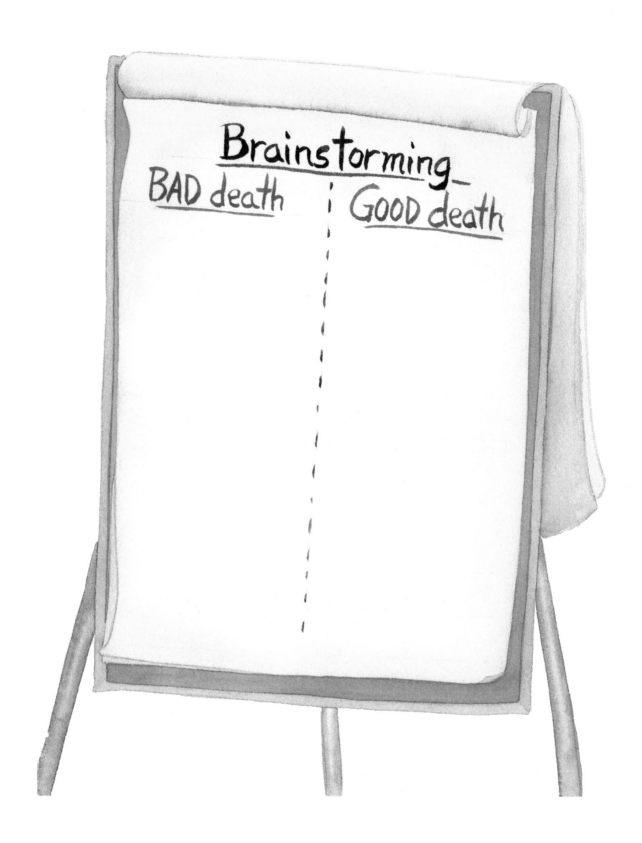

15. In the space below reflect on the concept of roadblocks to communication as identified on pages 37 to 40 of the text.

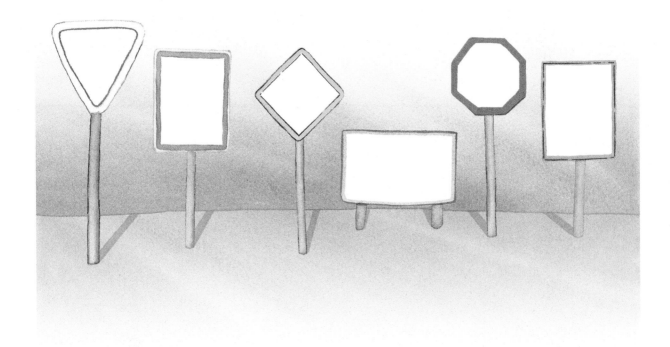

16. Reflect on ways to encourage open communication.

_____

_____

_____

_____

_____

_____

_____

_____

_____

_____

_____

_____

_____

_____

_____

_____

_____

_____

_____

_____

_____

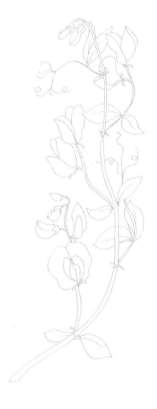

Increasing Physical Comfort

4

Understanding Your Beliefs and Baggage

1. Reflect on your experiences of pain, and reflect on your family's experiences of pain. Consider your beliefs about pain management. Did you grow up in a home in which family members were comfortable with using medications to manage pain, or do you come from a home in which family members opposed the use of medications? Reflect on and write about this.

_____

_____

_____

_____

_____

_____

_____

_____

_____

_____

_____

_____

_____

Solidifying Concepts

PSWs are directly and closely involved with all aspects of a dying person's everyday care. In addition, PSWs see the person much more—and more realistically—than other members of the health care team and so must also be the "eyes and ears" of others involved, noting and sharing information that may be useful to them.

2. Complete the crossword puzzle on physical care and comfort measures below.

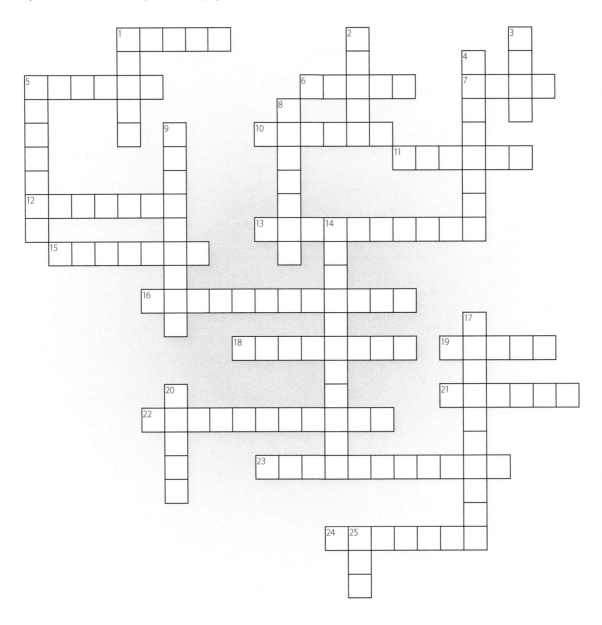

Across

1. Choose care strategies that best meet the _____ of the dying person at this time with this symptom.

5. After administering medications, monitor, _____, and report the person's responses.

6. Family may mistakenly believe that starting opioid medications for their loved one means that _____ is imminent.

7. _____ delivery is the most common route for giving medication. It is also the simplest.

10. People taking opioids may experience a number of side effects, including constipation and feeling nauseated, confused, and _____.

11. Family may be concerned that their loved one will become an _____ if they take opioids.

12. In a long-term care facility you might find clues to what _____ measures to use by looking at the person's shelves, walls, and trinkets.

13. Gathering information using the List of Sample Questions will help you to _____ize comfort measures to the person.

15. _____ is a program of care for the dying.

16. A _____ dose may be needed to manage pain between regular medication doses.

18. Since its beginning, the hospice _____ has spread worldwide.

19. Using items in the comfort basket may help a person _____ while they wait for medications to take effect.

21. It is important for the team to educate the _____ so that they can participate in providing care.

22. The Palliative Performance Scale (PPS) helps caregivers understand a person's level of _____.

23. The _____ decides the goal for pain relief. (2 words)

24. Medications called _____ are used when managing moderate to severe pain.

Down

1. Encourage the person and family to share their concerns about medications with the _____ or physician.

2. It is important to focus on the person's _____ of care when using palliation.

3. The sentiment "It's not being dead but the dying I _____" has been expressed by more than a few dying people.

4. Hospice care can be provided to a person in their home, the community, a _____, or a long-term care facility.

5. When providing comfort measures it is especially important to _____ the individual and individualize the care.

8. One principle of palliation is to _____ the symptom whenever possible.

9. In the PPS, intake is scaled from normal intake to reduced, to minimal to sips, to _____ only. (2 words)

14. PSWs might use the List of Sample Questions to gather _____.

17. The PPS is used to observe key indicators and _____ in order to understand a person's level of functioning.

20. Playing carefully chosen _____ can successfully distract a person from pain, reduce their anxiety or agitation, and promote sleep.

25. Mobility level, evidence of disease, activity level, ability for self-care, intake, and level of consciousness are used to determine a person's _____.

(Answer key is on page 59.)

3. Caregivers in many work settings use the Palliative Performance Scale (PPS) to identify the dying person's current level of functioning and needs, changes, and the need to adapt the care plan. What five things are measured on the scale?

   a. _____

   b. _____

   c. _____

   d. _____

   e. _____

4. Describe a person's level of functioning when they have a PPS of 20%.

   _____

   _____

   _____

5. Describe a person's level of functioning when they have a PPS of 10%.

   _____

   _____

   _____

6. As a PSW, you may advocate for the person and/or their family. Below, circle the options that are within your scope of practice.

   a. Offer information brochures to the family to clarify services.

   b. Share your concerns about the person's level of comfort at their care conference.

   c. Suggest that the family list their concerns, questions, and goals of care to refer to when they talk with the physician.

   d. Advise the family to increase the person's pain medication.

7. Circle the principles of palliation that guide the health care team when managing symptoms.

   a. Focus on the person's goals of care.

   b. Use nonpharmacological comfort measures when possible.

   c. Use medications to manage symptoms only when death is imminent.

   d. Monitor, record, and report the person's responses to medications and other comfort measures.

8. Circle the principles that guide the ordering and administration of medications in HPC.

    a. The health care team determines the goal for pain relief.

    b. Medications should only be given after pain occurs, not on a regular schedule.

    c. Breakthrough doses are used when a symptom recurs between regularly scheduled doses.

    d. A combination of medications may be necessary to control a symptom and side effects.

    e. Side effects and fears or concerns about medications should be recorded and reported.

    f. Nonpharmacological comfort measures may help improve comfort.

9. Opioids are commonly used to help manage pain and difficulty breathing.

True   **False**   (circle your answer)

10. These are the four most common side effects of opioids (circle your answer):

    a. Nausea/vomiting, drowsiness, addiction, confusion

    b. Nausea/vomiting, drowsiness, confusion, insomnia

    c. Constipation, addiction, nausea/vomiting, confusion

    d. Nausea/vomiting, constipation, drowsiness, confusion

11. The most common concerns people have about using opioids are constipation and addiction.

True   **False**   (circle your answer)

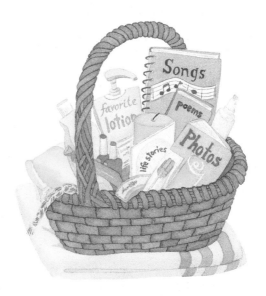

Bowel Function

12. Complete the table below.

How you might help prevent constipation	What you might observe if a person is constipated	What you might ask a dying person to better understand their needs	Comfort measures that might be helpful
1.	1.	1.	1.
2.	2.	2.	2.
3.	3.	3.	3.

Decreased Appetite and Weight Loss

13. Read "Profound Truths of Nutrition" on page 72 in the text. Explain these truths in your own words as if you were talking with a member of your own family.

_____

_____

_____

_____

14. The dying person often loses both weight and interest in eating. Refer to the story of Yetta on page 17 in the text. What did Yetta do to address her lack of appetite? Identify five things that you, as a PSW, could have done to help Yetta and her family adjust to her decrease in appetite.

_____

_____

_____

_____

_____

Dehydration

15. Read pages 74 to 76 in the text. Complete the table below.

What you might observe if a person is dehydrated	What you might ask a dying person to better understand their needs	Comfort measures that might be helpful
1.	1.	1.
2.	2.	2.
3.	3.	3.

Delirium

16. Mrs. Marsh is a resident at your hospice. You are called by Mrs. Marsh's daughter, who is very concerned about recent behaviour changes in her mother that include pacing, inability to carry on a conversation, and refusing to take medication.

Complete the table below.

What you might observe if a person has delirium	What you might ask a dying person to better understand their needs	Comfort measures that might be helpful
1.	1.	1.
2.	2.	2.
3.	3.	3.

Difficulty Breathing

17. Complete the exercise below to experience dyspnea.

Dyspnea Exercise

Materials: Three disposable drinking straws

Location: A place with room to walk

Note: People with respiratory or heart problems should not participate in this exercise.

Exercise:

   a. Compress the end of one straw and insert it into the end of a second straw.

   b. Compress the end of the third straw and insert it into one end of the double straw to form an extra-long straw.

   c. Pinch your nostrils to cut off airflow through them.

   d. Place the straw in your mouth and begin breathing through it.

   e. Walk around for two minutes.

   f. At the end of two minutes, remove the straw from your mouth and stop plugging your nose. Take a moment to allow your breathing and sensations to return to normal.

You have just experienced sensations similar to those that people with dyspnea have.

Answer the following questions:

a. What did the experience feel like? Describe it.

_____

_____

_____

b. What were your thoughts as the exercise progressed?

_____

_____

_____

c. How do feel you would respond if that sensation happened to you suddenly? What would you think was happening?

_____

_____

_____

18. Complete the table below.

How you might prevent difficulty breathing	What you might observe if a person has difficulty breathing	What you might ask a dying person to better understand their needs	Comfort measures that might be helpful
1.	1.	1.	1.
2.	2.	2.	2.
3.	3.	3.	3.

Fatigue

19. If the person you are caring for has a PPS of 40% and is very fatigued, what comfort strategies can you suggest that might help them have the energy to accomplish their priority activities? Complete the table below.

How you might prevent fatigue	What you might ask a dying person to better understand their needs	Comfort measures that might be helpful
1.	1.	1.
2.	2.	2.
3.	3.	3.

Mouth Discomfort

20. Complete the table below.

What you might observe if a person has a dry mouth	What you might ask a dying person to better understand their needs	Comfort measures that might be helpful
1.	1.	1.
2.	2.	2.
3.	3.	3.

Nausea and Vomiting

21. Consider this scenario.

She was crying on the bed when I entered her room.

She said, "I'm so tired of this nausea; I wish I could just die."

I sat with her and held her hand. It was all I could think of to help at that moment.

When she was less distressed, we talked. I asked her what made the nausea worse and what made it better. We made a few changes and then I phoned the nurse to report.

a. Select and adapt questions from the List of Sample Questions on page 52 in the text that can help you gather information, figure out comfort measures that would be most helpful, and report to the nurse.

_____

_____

_____

_____

_____

b. Imagine the person's responses to your questions and write the notes that you would use to give a verbal report to the nurse.

_____

_____

_____

_____

_____

c. Write what you would document in the chart regarding this person's nausea.

_____

_____

_____

_____

Pain

22. Role-Play Exercise 1 (pages 33–34)

One participant takes the role of the PSW, and a second participant takes the role of the dying person, Mr. B, who is in pain. A third participant, preferably the instructor if available, takes the role of the nurse to whom the PSW reports.

In the role-play, Mr. B describes his pain to the PSW, using the information on page 34 provided for that role.

The PSW gathers information about Mr. B by asking him questions based on the List of Sample Questions on page 52 in the text, and records the information in Mr. B's chart (page 33). Using that information, the PSW prepares a report for the nurse and presents it to the nurse orally.

Marking sheets for this exercise are provided on pages 60 and 61 of this workbook, in the appendix. The participants may find the marking sheets will help them in playing their part.

23. Change roles and complete Role-Play Exercise 2 (pages 35–36).

PSW Role

Mr. B is 75 years old. He has prostate cancer and is dying. He lives alone. You visit Mr. B in his home daily to assist him with personal care, remind him to take his medications, and set out a meal.

Usually he is very happy to see you and he loves to talk. Today he acknowledges your arrival but only mutters a response when you greet him. His dinner plate from last night is on the table and the food was not eaten. When you ask him how he is, he says he did not sleep last night, is in pain, and can hardly move because his left hip is so sore. He says he is tired of being sick. When you suggest a bath, he says that there is no way that he can even get to the bathroom.

You realize Mr. B's condition has changed and that you need to record your observations of his pain, report to the nurse, and ask the nurse for help to develop a new plan for his care today. You remember the List of Sample Questions that you can adapt to use in obtaining the information that you will need to provide an excellent report for the nurse. You have the list in your backpack, so you get it out and ask Mr. B. the questions that will help you provide enough information to the nurse.

Mr. B. is able to answer all of your questions; you just need to remember what to ask him.

Complete the following:

a. Adapt the List of Sample Questions on page 52 in the text to help you gather information about Mr. B's pain.

_____

_____

_____

b. Record your observations in Mr. B's "chart" (below).

_____

_____

_____

c. Prepare an oral report and deliver it to the nurse.

_____

_____

_____

d. Discuss what you learned in this exercise with your role-play partner.

Person in Pain "Mr. B" Role

A PSW comes to see you every day. Today you are particularly pleased to see the PSW because you are really in a lot of pain and need help.

When the PSW asks you about your pain, you provide information as described below.

Do not volunteer information unless the PSW asks you for it.

The pain started yesterday, after you fell on the way to the kitchen. The neighbour was there and helped you back to bed. You figure that you hurt your hip when you fell; it has been aching ever since. The aching will not stop. It is the worst pain you have had since getting sick and almost as bad as when you broke your leg 20 years ago.

The medications that you take five times a day help you feel a bit better but only for an hour or so. Your neighbour gave you a cold pack, but you can't get out of bed to get it. Rubbing your hip helps a bit.

Rating your pain, you figure it is a 7 out of 10 on a scale of 1 to 10, on which 0 is no pain and 10 is the worst pain you can imagine. You couldn't sleep last night and feel exhausted. You are miserable and just want some help.

You are so glad that the PSW came and is so helpful.

PSW Role

Mr. K has lived on the unit where you work for two years. He is 85 years old and has osteoporosis and a history of multiple fractures. Mr. K. is cognitively able and alert, but is very frail and slow moving.

Today when you help him get up he is really hesitant to move and gets out of bed very carefully. When you comment on his slow movements and his apparent stiffness, he says that he is in pain and that he can hardly move because his back is so sore. He says he did not sleep much last night. He is willing to get up to sit in the chair by the bed but does not want to go to the dining room for breakfast. He is very worried about his back.

You realize Mr. K's condition has changed and that you need to record your observations of his pain, report to the nurse, and ask the nurse for help to develop a new plan for his care today. You remember the List of Sample Questions that you can adapt to use in obtaining the information that you will need to provide an excellent report for the nurse. You have the list in your backpack, so you get it out and ask Mr. K. the questions that will help you provide enough information to the nurse.

Mr. K. is able to answer all of your questions; you just need to remember what to ask him.

Complete the following:

a. Adapt the List of Sample Questions on page 52 in the text to help you gather information about Mr. K's pain.

_____

_____

_____

b. Record your observations in Mr. K's "chart" (below).

_____

_____

_____

c. Prepare an oral report and deliver it to the nurse.

_____

_____

_____

d. Discuss what you learned in this exercise with your role-play partner.

Person in Pain "Mr. K" Role

Your PSW comes to help you get out of bed today. You wish the PSW would take care of everyone else first, because you are so sore! Your back hurts worse than it has for ages!

When the PSW asks you questions about your pain, provide the information as described below.

Do not volunteer information unless the PSW asks you for it.

The pain really increased during the night. You don't know what happened to cause it to get so bad. You are worried that you have another fracture. You hope the doctor will come see you and check it out.

The pain is worse than the other pains you have had before. This one is terrible! In fact, if they ask you to rate the pain, you might even say this pain rates 8 out of 10 on a scale of 1 to 10, on which 0 is no pain and 10 is the worst pain you can imagine. It hurts in your upper and lower back, and the sharp and shooting pain goes down your legs.

You take only the regular medications that the nurse gives you every morning and at lunch and suppertime.

You wish your wife were alive, because she would help you by giving you a warm flannel blanket.

You wish you could just stay in bed and not get up, and you definitely do not want to go to breakfast.

24. Complete the table below.

What you might observe if a person has pain/discomfort	What you might ask a dying person to better understand their needs	Comfort measures that might be helpful
1.	1.	1.
2.	2.	2.
3.	3.	3.

25. Refer to the story about Annette on page 108 in the text.

a. How did the PSW identify Annette's pain?

_____

_____

_____

b. What did the PSW do to help address Annette's pain?

_____

_____

_____

c. Write a verbal report to share information with the nurse about Annette.

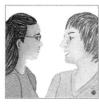

_____

_____

_____

_____

_____

_____

d. Follow-up after giving medication is as important as the original charting to report pain. Write a sample chart entry following up on Annette.

charting

Providing Psychosocial Care

5

Understanding Your Beliefs and Baggage

1. Refer to pages 36 to 46 in the text and identify good communication practices that you already use.

_____

_____

_____

_____

2. Recall a time when someone shared a painful experience with you and you wanted to help fix the problem. Think about that time and your response. What part of your response suggests that you were in the Fix-It Trap?

_____

_____

_____

_____

_____

_____

3. This exercise is designed to help you understand the importance of helping people with life-threatening illnesses determine their priorities and maintain their choices.

   a. In the large box below, write all of the things that are important to you in your life (e.g., people, activities, events, foods).

   b. In the medium-sized box, write about what you would do if you had only three months to live.

   c. In the small circle, write about what you would do if you had only three days to live.

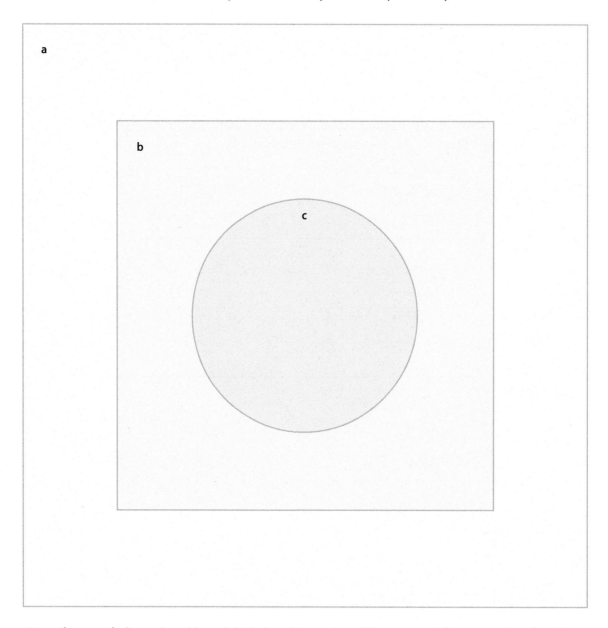

Note: If you are feeling vulnerable and think that this exercise will be too much for you, work with a colleague or the instructor to adapt this activity to meet your needs. If this exercise triggers strong responses, consider debriefing with a colleague or the instructor.

Now think about your responses to the exercise and do some reflective writing guided by the questions below:

d. What were your feelings as you wrote in the large box? The medium box? The small circle? What thoughts do you associate with these feelings?

_____

_____

_____

_____

_____

_____

_____

e. Write about your decision-making process on what to write in the shapes. Did you change your mind? How did you make a final decision?

_____

_____

_____

_____

_____

_____

f. How would you feel if you were not able to do what you wrote in the circle?

_____

_____

_____

_____

_____

_____

4. Reflect on this story and answer the questions below it.

You have been assisting a man with personal care regularly for several months. You have become very fond of him and his partner and enjoy providing care. When you arrive today, the partner informs you that the person has decided not to continue with kidney dialysis. The doctors suggest that without dialysis he might have a few weeks to live. You realize that this will shorten his life significantly.

a. What feelings, thoughts, and questions might you have?

_____

_____

_____

b. With whom is it appropriate to discuss your questions and feelings?

_____

_____

c. How can you show respect for the man's decision and his right to make his own decisions? How can you control your facial expressions so that you do not share your judgment with the man or his family?

_____

_____

_____

_____

d. What might you say to or do for the person you are caring for?

_____

_____

_____

Solidifying Concepts

5. Write five things you learned about grief that you did not know before reading the text.

_____

_____

_____

_____

_____

6. Review page 129 in the text and fill in the blanks in the paragraph below.

Advance care planning is about the _____ that people have with

_____ and _____ about their

_____, _____ and _____.

It is the process of _____, in the event that you _____,

_____, or _____.

7. Review pages 129 to 130 in the text and fill in the blanks in the sentences below.

a. A _____ is chosen by the person or the health care team to speak on

behalf of the person in the event that the person is no longer able to direct his or her own care.

b. When a _____ is making health care decisions, they must be based on what

the _____ wants, not based on what the _____

would want for herself or himself.

8. The PSW can sign documents, including wills, legal forms, and contracts.

True   **False**   (circle your answer)

9. Complete the crossword puzzle on psychosocial issues below.

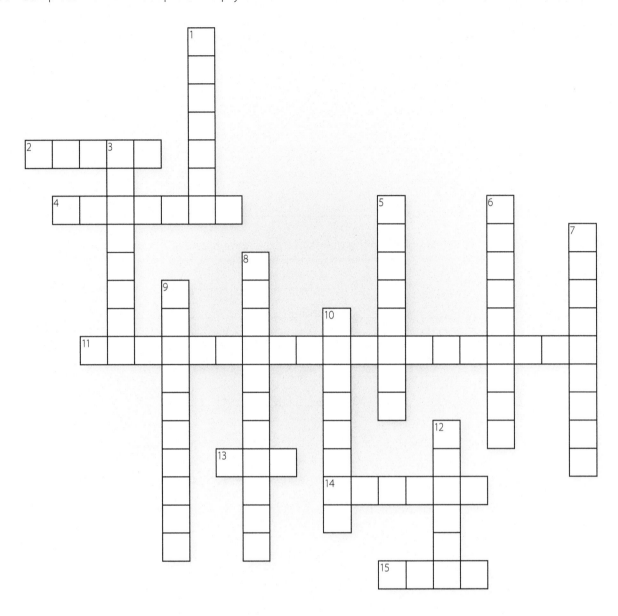

Across

2. _____ is our response to loss.

4. The role of the PSW is to provide _____.

11. It is important for people to have conversations about what is important to them and what care they want if they become unable to speak for themselves. These conversations are part of _____. (3 words)

13. The role of the PSW is not to _____ problems.

14. Loss and grief are _____ parts of life.

15. We experience _____ when someone or something important to us is no longer available.

Down

1. The _____ is responsible for reviewing sudden deaths.

3. Preparing mentally and emotionally for an _____ loss can make it easier to manage.

5. A person with a life-threatening illness and declining health experiences _____ losses.

6. _____ questions provide the opportunity for the person to explore their feelings. (2 words)

7. Losses that are not clearly defined, such as those experienced by people with dementia, are considered to be _____.

8. One of the psychosocial issues that dying people face is living with _____.

9. Examples of _____ to communication include offering praise, false reassurance, and advice.

10. _____ is the process a person goes through after losing someone or something.

12. Hospice palliative care specialists no longer believe that people grieve in specific _____.

(Answer key is on page 62.)

Integrating into Practice

10. Complete the exercise below to learn about your personal responses to loss.

Multiple Losses Exercise

On each of six pieces of paper, write down one activity that you enjoy (writing lightly with the pencil will decrease the chance of the writing being legible from the reverse side of the paper when it is turned over). Lay the papers writing side down on the table in front of you. Shuffle them around such that you no longer know which is which. Line them up in a row.

Turn over the middle two pieces of paper and imagine that because of declining health you are no longer able to do these activities. What is your immediate response to having these two activities removed from your life? What do you feel? What do you think?

_____

_____

_____

Resist the urge to change an activity that you lost to a different one. This exercise is designed to help you imagine the multiple losses that dying people experience.

Now imagine it is two weeks later and the doctor tells you that you should no longer do two more of the activities. What do you feel about these new losses? Do you feel better knowing that you still have two activities left?

_____

_____

_____

Now imagine that you wake one morning a month later and are unable to do the remaining two activities. What do you feel? What do you want to do or say?

_____

_____

_____

Discuss your experience with a colleague.

11. Review pages 138 to 140 in the text about grief being a whole person experience.

   a. Mark the illustration below using words, colours, and shapes to indicate how you experience grief and how it affects you physically, emotionally, spiritually, and socially.

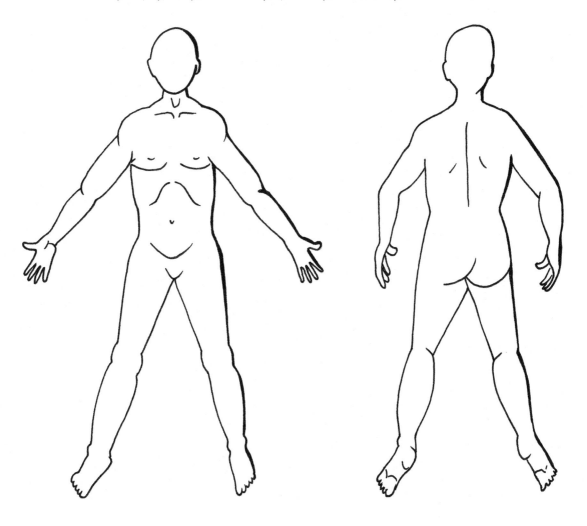

   b. Reflect on how grief is a whole person experience.

   _____

   _____

   _____

   _____

   _____

   _____

   _____

c. Think about a friend or family member who has experienced loss and grief in their life. Use the illustration below to create a picture of grief as you saw your friend or family member experience it.

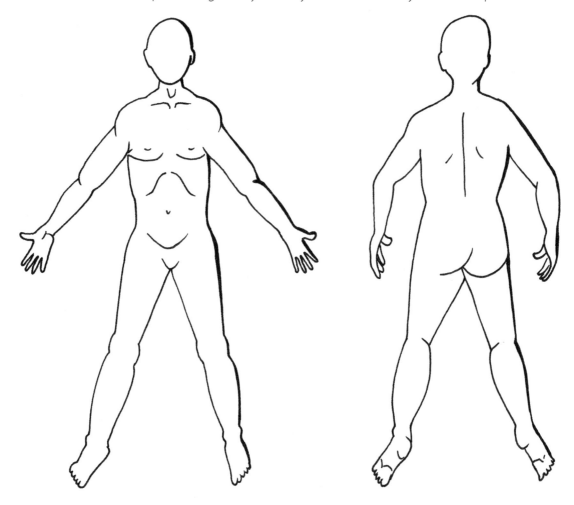

12. Identify five ways to support a grieving person.

_____

_____

_____

_____

_____

_____

_____

_____

Caring in the Last Days and Hours

6

Understanding Your Beliefs and Baggage

1. Reflect on and write about your feelings regarding caring for someone in their last days and hours and at the time of death. Compare this reflection to the feelings you identified, in exercise 3 in chapter 1 of this workbook, about working with people who are dying. Your feelings today may be similar to those you identified before or may have changed.

_____

_____

_____

_____

_____

_____

_____

_____

2. PSWs often provide care for a person's body after death has occurred. For some people this is a sacred ritual; others are not comfortable doing this. Reflect on how you feel about caring for the body after death. If you feel uncomfortable, consider asking a colleague or supervisor to mentor you and help you become more comfortable. You may want to ask for additional opportunities at work to gain experience providing this kind of care. Reflect on and write about caring for the body after death.

_____

_____

_____

_____

_____

_____

_____

_____

Solidifying Concepts

3. Refer to pages 160 to 167 in the text and complete the following chart.

Physical changes in the last days and hours	Comfort measures for the dying person	Comfort measures for the family
Decreased physical strength and increased drowsiness		
Reduced intake and difficulty swallowing		
Delirium or confusion		
Agitation or restlessness		
Unresponsiveness		
Irregular breathing		
Congested breathing		
Changes in skin colour and temperature		
Dry eyes		
Decreased urinary output		
Bowel or bladder incontinence		

4. What physical changes in a dying person suggest that death is very close?

_____

_____

_____

_____

5. You enter a person's room and notice that the person is not breathing. Create a list of tasks to complete if this occurred in a home setting and in a long-term care facility.

Home Setting

a. _____

b. _____

c. _____

d. _____

e. _____

f. _____

Long-term Care Facility

a. _____

b. _____

c. _____

d. _____

e. _____

f. _____

6. It is always important to know what a person's DNR status is before entering their home.

True   False   (circle your answer)

7. Describe four ways you can support the family after the death of their loved one.

a. _____

b. _____

c. _____

d. _____

8. List three ways you can you show respect and support for people whose cultural traditions or spiritual practices are different from yours.

a. _____

b. _____

c. _____

9. Review page 187 in the text, and fill in the blanks in the paragraph below.

When a person's death is sudden, unexpected, or occurs within 24 hours of admission to a hospital, the coroner is notified. The role of the coroner is to confirm the _____ of the person who died and the probable _____ and _____ of death. The coroner classifies the death as natural, accidental, suicide, homicide, or undetermined.

Integrating into Practice

10. Discuss the topics below in small groups or with a colleague.

   a. Different traditions and practices in caring for the body after death has occurred.

   b. Ways to support the family when they participate in a cultural practice that does not have meaning for you or seem necessary.

11. When you are at work or during a practicum, refer to the agency's or facility's policy and procedures manual and look up care of the body following death.

Caring for *You!*

7

Just as the health care team needs to individualize care to meet the needs of those they care for, each member of the health care team needs to personalize self-care strategies.

1. List, mind map, or draw activities that help you to refuel and re-energize.

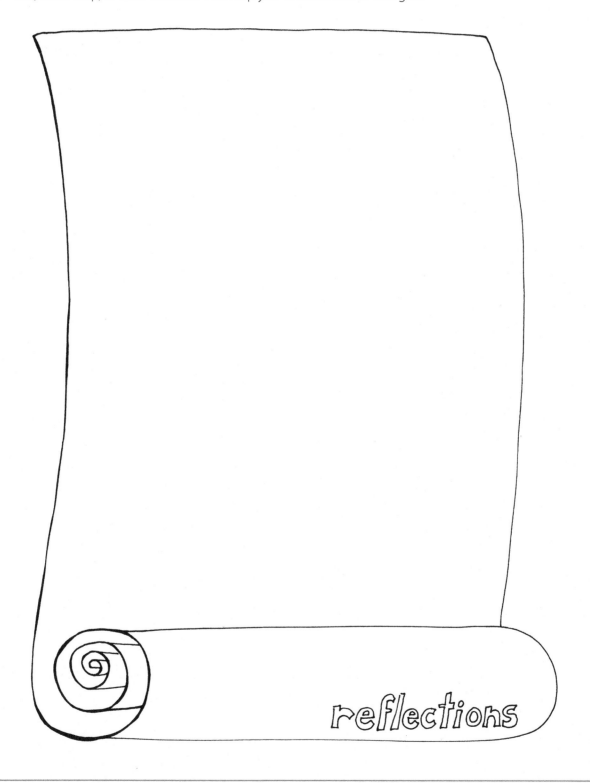

reflections

2. Reflect on the term "self-care." Write freely for five minutes about the topic of self-care. What did you learn? Where did your reflections take you?

_____

_____

_____

_____

_____

_____

_____

_____

_____

_____

_____

_____

_____

_____

_____

_____

_____

_____

_____

_____

_____

_____

3. Review the information about compassion fatigue in chapter 7 of the text.

    a. Write freely for five minutes about compassion fatigue.

_____

_____

_____

_____

_____

_____

_____

_____

_____

_____

_____

_____

_____

_____

_____

_____

_____

_____

_____

_____

b. Review the chart on pages 194 and 195 in the text. What zone are you in?

Red   Green   Yellow   (circle your answer)

c. Respond to the reflection questions in the table that relate to the zone you are in.

_____

_____

_____

_____

_____

_____

_____

_____

_____

4. Self-care can be integrated into your working life. The story on page 179 of the text describes a difficult death. Following the death, the PSW did a few key things that not only helped the family, but also probably left her feeling more at peace with the death and more satisfied with the care she provided. Read the story and identify what the PSW did that benefited both the family and herself.

_____

_____

_____

_____

_____

_____

_____

_____

_____

_____

5. Education is one of the finest forms of self-care! The books, movies, and websites listed below are about dying, death, hospice palliative care, and caregiving. They were chosen because they are classics, thought-provoking, or just plain good

   a. Circle titles that interest you.

      Albom, M. *Tuesdays with Morrie: An Old Man, a Young Man, and Life's Greatest Lesson.* New York: Random House, 1997.

      Buckman, R. *I Don't Know What to Say: How to Help and Support Someone Who Is Dying.* Toronto: Key Porter Books, 2005.

      Callanan, M., and P. Kelley. *Final Gifts: Understanding the Special Awareness, Needs, and Communications of the Dying.* Toronto: Bantam Books, 1993.

      Joseph, E. *In the Slender Margin: The Intimate Strangeness of Dying.* Toronto: HarperCollins, 2014. (This book is a journey into the land of death and dying seen through the lens of art and the imagination.)

      Mathieu, F. *The Compassion Fatigue Workbook.* New York: Routledge, 2012.

      O'Rourke, M., and E. Dufour. *Embracing the End of Life: Help for Those Who Accompany the Dying.* Toronto: Novalis, 2012.

      Schwalbe, W. *The End of Your Life Book Club.* New York: First Vintage Books, 2012.

   b. Circle movies that you want to see.

      A Story about Care (15-minute video, available on Vimeo at http://vimeo.com/57786711, or Canadian Virtual Hospice, www.virtualhospice.ca).

      Empathy: The Human Connection to Patient Care
      (4-minute video, available on YouTube at http://youtu.be/cDDWvj_q-o8)

      The Bucket List (2007, Jack Nicholson, Morgan Freeman. Two terminally ill men who meet as patients in a hospital head off with a list of things they want to do before they die.)

      Wit (2001, Emma Thompson. A professor reassesses her life when she finds out she has terminal ovarian cancer.)

   c. Circle websites that you want to explore.

      Canadian Hospice Palliative Care Association, www.chpca.net

      Canadian Virtual Hospice, www.virtualhospice.ca

      Life and Death Matters, www.lifeanddeathmatters.ca

      Speak Up: Advance Care Planning in Canada, www.advancecareplanning.ca

      The Way Forward: An Integrated Palliative Approach to Care, www.hpcintegration.ca

      Your provincial hospice palliative care association

6. Consider what you have learned while studying hospice palliative care. Reflect on and write about your learning and then discuss the topics below in pairs or small groups.

    a. Your reflections on the text and workbook, the content, and the learning activities

    _____

    _____

    _____

    b. What you want to learn more about, and what you would change or add or delete

    _____

    _____

    _____

    c. Three things that you learned about integrating a palliative approach that you want to integrate into your practice

    _____

    _____

    _____

7. Take 5 or 10 minutes as you finish this workbook and explore self-care in your life. What commitment can you make to yourself to take care of *you*?

    _____

    _____

    _____

    _____

    _____

    _____

    _____

Appendix

Answers to Hospice Palliative Care puzzle, page 12

Across

2. team
4. quality
7. community
8. diagnosis
9. end of life
10. Saunders
12. volunteer
14. residential
15. symptom
16. normal
17. communicate
19. Hospice
23. bereavement
25. unit
26. affirms
27. grief

Down

1. holistic
3. approach
5. boundaries
6. long term care
11. listen
13. disease
18. care
20. scope
21. cancer
22. settings
24. nurse

Answers to Physical Care puzzle, page 22

Across

1. needs
5. record
6. death
7. Oral
10. drowsy
11. addict
12. comfort
13. individual
15. Hospice
16. breakthrough
18. movement
19. relax
21. family
22. functioning
23. dying person
24. opioids

Down

1. nurse
2. goals
3. fear
4. hospital
5. respect
8. prevent
9. mouth care
14. information
17. behaviours
20. music
25. PPS

Marking Sheet for the Role-Play Exercises on Pain*

*The group, not individual students, will be marked.

Students in group: _____

Exercise (circle number):   1   2

Role-Play	Possible Marks	Comments
Student playing the person in pain	1	
Student playing the person in pain describes it using the information provided	1	
Student playing the PSW adapts the List of Sample Questions (see below) and gathers needed information		
What is happening? What is wrong?	1	
When did it start?	1	
Where do you feel it?	1	
How does it feel?	1	
Can you rate it on a scale? 0 to 10 (0 = no symptom and 10 = the worst imaginable) Small, medium, large Mild, moderate, severe	1	
What makes it better or worse?	1	
What would be helpful? What can I do to help you?	1	
What do you want to see/have happen?	1	
Nurse receives a clear and complete report from the PSW		
Record/documentation is clear, concise, and accurately reflects the verbal report.	1	
The reporting is free of judgments and focuses on key information.	1	
The students reflect on their learning experience and how they can apply it in practice.	3	
TOTAL MARKS GIVEN	**/15**	

Marking Sheet for the Role-Play Exercises on Pain*

*The group, not individual students, will be marked.

Students in group: _____

Exercise (circle number):　　　　1　　　　2

Role-Play	Possible Marks	Comments
Student playing the person in pain	1	
Student playing the person in pain describes it using the information provided	1	
Student playing the PSW adapts the List of Sample Questions (see below) and gathers needed information		
What is happening? What is wrong?	1	
When did it start?	1	
Where do you feel it?	1	
How does it feel?	1	
Can you rate it on a scale? 0 to 10 (0 = no symptom and 10 = the worst imaginable) Small, medium, large Mild, moderate, severe	1	
What makes it better or worse?	1	
What would be helpful? What can I do to help you?	1	
What do you want to see/have happen?	1	
Nurse receives a clear and complete report from the PSW		
Record/documentation is clear, concise, and accurately reflects the verbal report.	1	
The reporting is free of judgments and focuses on key information.	1	
The students reflect on their learning experience and how they can apply it in practice.	3	
TOTAL MARKS GIVEN	**/15**	

Answers to Psychosocial Issues puzzle, page 44

Across

2. Grief

4. support

11. advance care planning

13. fix

14. normal

15. loss

Down

1. coroner

3. expected

5. multiple

6. Open ended

7. ambiguous

8. uncertainty

9. roadblocks

10. Grieving

12. stages

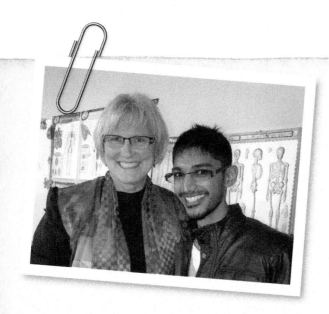

Please feel free to email me your reflections. I so appreciate receiving feedback and stories.

May you feel more comfortable, be more competent, and provide excellent care for the dying and their families. And may your work enrich and bless your life.

Warm regards,
Kath Murray

CPSIA information can be obtained
at www.ICGtesting.com
Printed in the USA
LVOW05s1824060816

499318LV00004B/6/P